BEAUTIFUL
BRAIDS

BEAUTIFUL

BRAIDS

Easy, Elegant Looks
For Braided Hair

JAMES TAKOS WITH KARIN STROM

PHOTOGRAPHY BY RICHARD DILLON/OZ: NEW YORK

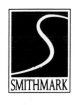

A FRIEDMAN GROUP BOOK

© 1994 by Michael Friedman Publishing Group, Inc.

This edition published in 1994 by SMITHMARK Publishers Inc. 16 East 32nd Street, New York, NY 10016.

SMITHMARK books are available for bulk purchase for sales promotion and premium use. For details, write or call the manager of special sales, SMITHMARK Publishers Inc., 16 East 32nd Street, New York, NY 10016; (212) 532-6600.

ISBN 0-8317-0991-X

BEAUTIFUL BRAIDS
Easy, Elegant Looks for Braided Hair
was prepared and produced by
Michael Friedman Publishing Group, Inc.
15 West 26th Street
New York NY 10010

Art Director: Jeff Batzli
Designer: Judy Morgan
Photography Director: Christopher C. Bain

Typeset by Classic Type, Inc.
Color separations by Universal Colour Scanning Ltd.
Printed and bound in China by Leefung-Asco Printers Ltd.

10 9 8 7 6 5 4 3 2 1

With love and thanks to the people from "Oz": Timothy, Sally, Mari, and Boda. I couldn't have done it without you.

C O N T E N T S

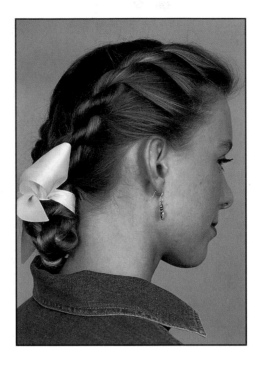

CONTENTS

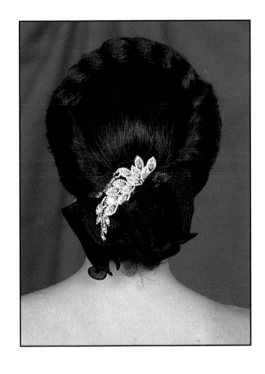

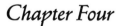

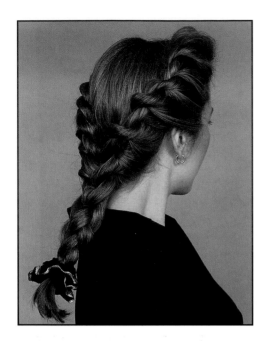

Beautiful Braids will allow you to say good-bye to the notion that braids are just a way that young girls keep hair off their faces while they are playing. Since ancient times, hair braids have been used not only as practical tools for managing long hair, but also as beautiful decoration. Braids can provide a woman with an infinite variety of looks with a minimum of time and effort. And they can accommodate any woman's style: a simple topknot is the perfect accompaniment to a sleek tailored suit; a French braid with wisps and bangs allowed to peek out can work perfectly with jeans and a sweater; and an elegant French twist will add special glamour to an evening gown.

Beautiful Braids makes a wonderful variety of braided hairstyles that look as if they were done by a professional hairdresser accessible to any woman. In the first three chapters, it provides directions and illustrations for executing the fundamental types of braids: basic braids, simple French braids, and rope braids. Each chapter also includes a wealth of variations, from a Basic Braid Dressed Up to a French-Braided Hairband to a Rope Braid to Bun. In chapter four, *Beautiful Braids* provides a variety of elegant styles that will add sophistication to any evening outfit. Although many of the designs look like they took hours and hours—or the help of a professional stylist—to achieve, they are surprisingly easy to do. Also included in this book are styles for kids' braids that will allow young girls to fix their own hair in wonderful ways right alongside Mom or big sister.

Although long hair offers the most possibilities for braids, women with medium-length hair will find that they too have a wide variety of braiding options. And even women with quite short hair can create many of the styles shown in this book with the use of a switch, a long hairpiece in the form of a removable ponytail, which is made of synthetic or human hair and is gathered at the top with a loop for easy attaching. Although you may be apprehensive about using switches at first, you are sure to find them fun to work with and to have your repertory of hair styles greatly expanded. Just be sure that when purchasing a switch, you match your own hair color and texture as closely as possible.

PREPARING YOUR SWITCH

Either have a friend hold the looped end of the switch securely or attach the loop to the back of a stable chair. Brush the hair until it is smooth, removing any tangles. For styles calling for a braided switch, divide into three equal sections and follow instructions for basic braiding (see page 11). For styles calling for a roped switch, divide the switch into two equal sections and follow

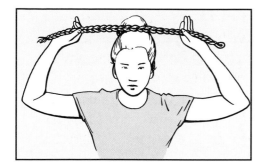

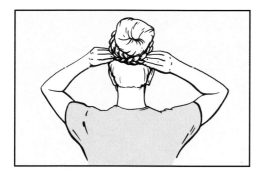

the instructions for roping (see page 37).

To attach the switch to your own hair, put a bobby pin through the loop at the end of the switch. (Your hair should already be in a ponytail.) Take the bobby pin and pin it securely through the covered elastic that is binding the ponytail. If necessary, use a second bobby pin to assure that the switch is firmly attached to your own hair.

TIPS

Whether you are working with a hairpiece or not, there are a few basic guidelines that will make your adventures in braiding go more smoothly.

❖ Always work with clean hair that has been brushed through and detangled.

❖ Very fine, limp hair can be set and dried to create more body.

❖ To help control flyaway hair, use a spritzer of water. If you have stubborn ends that insist on sticking out, smooth them down with gel.

❖ Be sure to have the proper tools on hand:

    A good hair brush
    A rat tail comb
    Bobby pins and hairpins to match your hair color
    A good supply of covered elastics (keep your eyes open for the really thick ones   they're hard to find)
    A spritzer
    Hair spray and gel
    Hair ornament, scrungies, barrettes, and/or ribbons

❖ When braiding, be sure to maintain even tension throughout. This is probably the most important rule of all. It applies to both the loose braids that tend to look more casual and to tighter, more controlled braiding. As you braid, a slight twist of each strand to the outside tends to give the style a neat, smooth look.

❖ Never give in to the temptation to use non-covered elastics on your hair. It is a guaranteed way to break ends and create hair havoc!

❖ Don't feel intimidated by the more difficult-looking styles—you can always enlist the help of a friend. This is a good way to become comfortable with the steps of a style. Then you'll be ready to try it on your own.

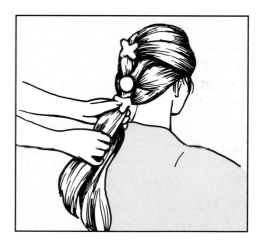

❖ Most important, enjoy experimenting with your hair. Once you've learned the basic techniques of braiding, French braiding, and roping, you're on your way. You may even get so good that you can design some styles of your own!

Chapter One

BASIC BRAIDS & TOPKNOTS

❖ ❖ ❖

BASIC BRAID

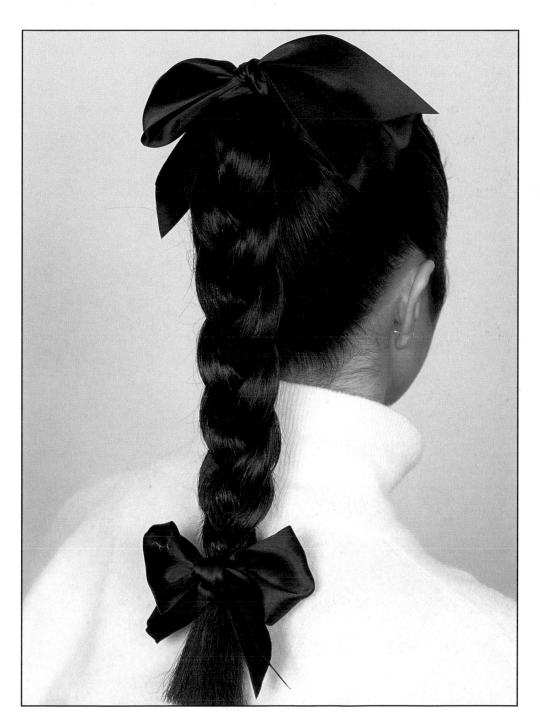

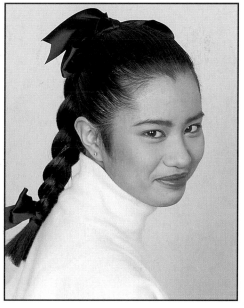

*i*f you've never braided hair before, you'll need to learn the Basic Braid first, for it is the technique used for many of the styles in this book. It is also a style of its own—it's cool, comfortable, neat, and easy. Practice until this technique is second nature to you, and it will serve as a springboard to the myriad of braids in these pages.

MATERIALS

2 covered elastic bands
2 double-face satin ribbons

DIRECTIONS

1. Sweep hair straight back into a high ponytail. Secure with a covered elastic band.

2. Divide ponytail into 3 equal sections. Hold one section to the left with your left hand and another section to the right with your right hand. Let the center section hang freely.

3. To braid:

(a) Cross the left section over the center section so that it becomes the "new" center section.

(b) Release the new center and grab hold of the new left section with your left hand.

(c) Repeat steps a and b with the strand in your right hand.

4. Continue crossing alternate sides over the center section. When you reach the end of the ponytail, secure the braid with an elastic band.

5. Tie satin ribbon bows to the top and bottom of the braid, concealing the elastic bands.

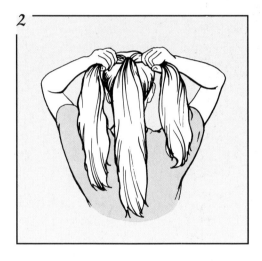

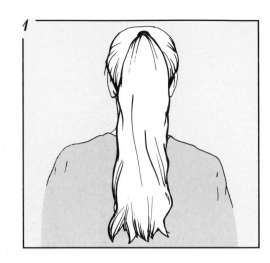

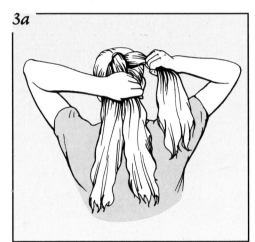

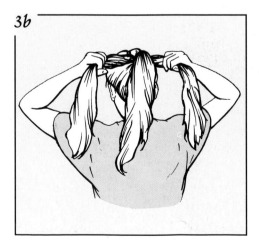

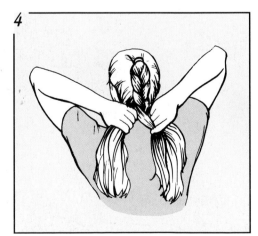

BASIC BRAID DRESSED UP

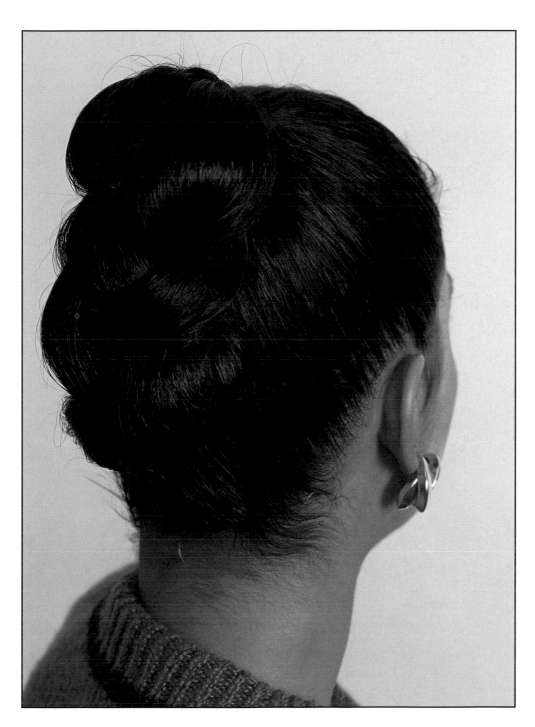

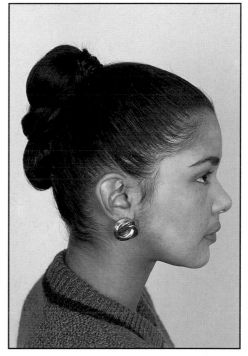

*h*ere's a simple way to dress up the Basic Braid. It is perfect for those days when you want to look special but don't have time to fuss. This style looks much more difficult than it really is, so it is a perfect next step for beginners. While some styles are best suited for certain types of hair, this one works well on straight or curly hair and hair of just about any length. You can tame short ends that won't stay in place with a curling iron and let them hang as tendrils around your face and at the nape of your neck.

MATERIALS

2 covered elastic bands
bobby pins   hairpins

DIRECTIONS

1. Sweep hair up into a high ponytail at the crown of your head. Secure with a covered elastic band. Section off a small strand (about ⅛ of total hair) from the underside of the ponytail.

2. Divide the small strand into three equal sections (**a**). Braid until you reach the end (**b**). You can simply twist this strand instead of braiding it if you prefer.

3. Wrap the long, skinny braid around the ponytail's elastic band. Secure the end of the braid with a bobby pin underneath the ponytail.

4. Loosely braid the main ponytail and secure the end with an elastic band.

5. Fold the long braid under at the nape of the neck and pin from underneath. Use hairpins along the sides of the braid to "invisibly" attach the braid to your head.

6. For a more casual look, loosen hair with the end of a rat tail comb.

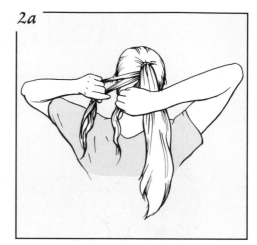

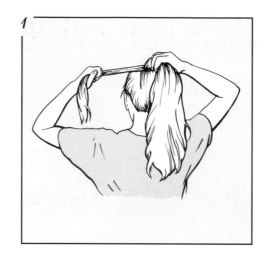

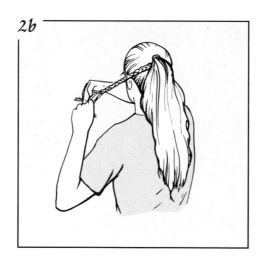

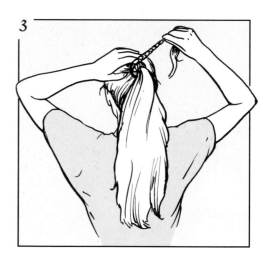

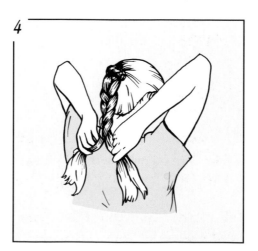

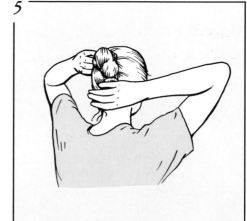

BRAIDED FIGURE EIGHT

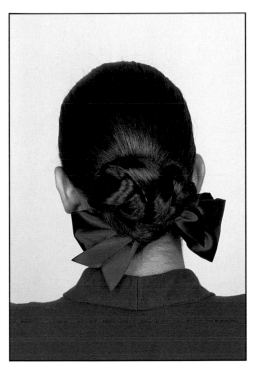

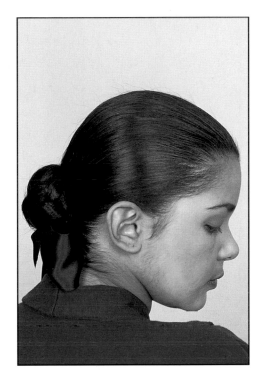

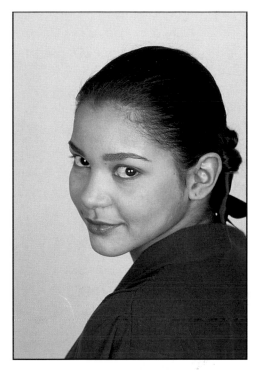

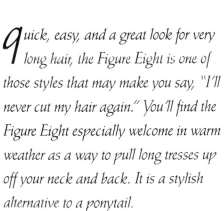

Quick, easy, and a great look for very long hair, the Figure Eight is one of those styles that may make you say, "I'll never cut my hair again." You'll find the Figure Eight especially welcome in warm weather as a way to pull long tresses up off your neck and back. It is a stylish alternative to a ponytail.

MATERIALS

2 covered elastic bands
ribbon
hairpins

DIRECTIONS

1. Sweep hair back into a ponytail at the nape of the neck and secure with a covered elastic band.

2. Braid the ponytail to the end and secure with a second elastic.

3. Tie a bow around the top elastic with a length of ribbon about twice as long as the braid. Cut the ends of the ribbon for neat, clean edges. Pull the bow around so it is underneath the braid.

4. To make a Figure Eight:
   (a) Hold the braid at the midpoint with your right hand. Twist it to the right one half-turn; you will feel the upper portion of the braid begin to "kink." Assist the kinking by pulling this portion up and to the left with your left hand. Fold this looped

braid flat against your head so the midpoint is at the center elastic. You have just formed the left loop of a sideways Figure Eight. You should have used half of the length of the braid. Anchor in place with hairpins.

(b) Twist the remaining half of the braid one half-turn to the right, folding it up to the right and down behind the bow. This completes the second loop of the sideways Figure Eight. Pin the end of the braid behind the back of the right side of the bow.

PRACTICE TIPS

Try this style first on a friend so you can see how the Figure Eight is formed. Soon you'll be able to do your own hair in this style simply by feel.

If you have difficulty getting the knack of it, try forming both sides of the Figure Eight before you add the hairpins. Leaving the loops free may help you master the folding technique as it allows you to move the braid around a little as you try to position it.

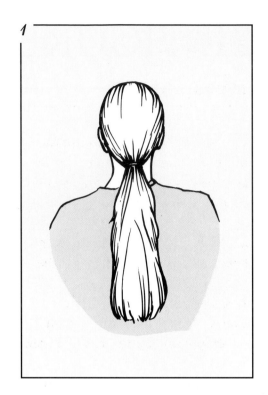

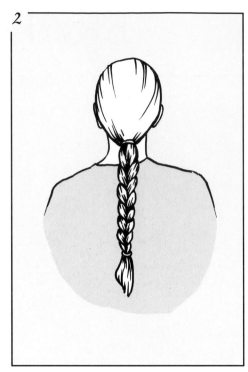

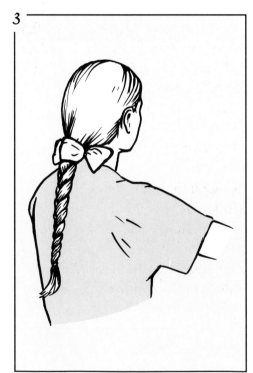

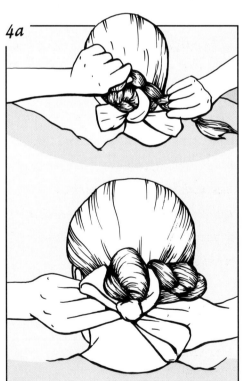

TOPKNOT

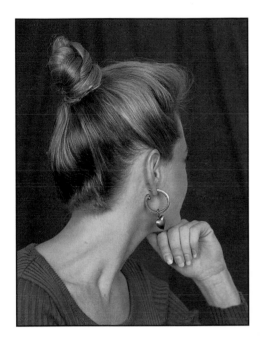

*t*he Topknot is a sophisticated look that can be both professional and chic. It takes almost no time to do and is the perfect way to deal with a "bad hair day"! Get in the habit of carrying some covered elastic bands in your purse (the chunky ones work best), and you can fashion a Topknot whenever you need to get your hair off your face. Hair gel keeps fly-away ends in place.

MATERIALS

2 covered elastic bands
bobby pins   hairpins

DIRECTIONS

1. Sweep all your hair except the front section into a ponytail at the crown of your head. Secure with a covered elastic band.

2. Sweep the front section back toward the ponytail and twist the end. Wrap the twisted section around the ponytail elastic to conceal it. Secure the end with a bobby pin underneath the ponytail.

3. Divide the ponytail into two sections. Twist each strand clockwise (hold each end securely so that the strands don't untwist) and then twine the twisted strands around each other. Secure with an elastic band.

4. Twist the rope clockwise.

5. Coil the twisted rope (also in a clockwise direction) around the base of the ponytail to shape the topknot. Secure with hairpins. Tuck any loose ends into the topknot, using gel if necessary.

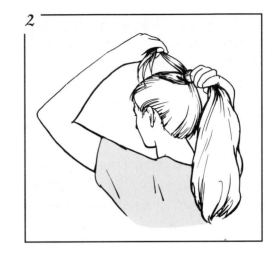

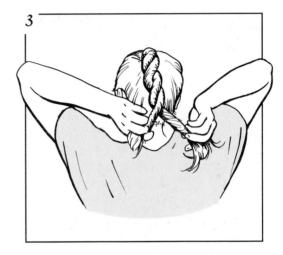

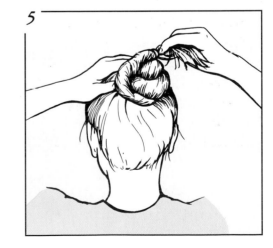

HIGH-VOLUME TOPKNOT WITH SINGLE-BRAID WRAP

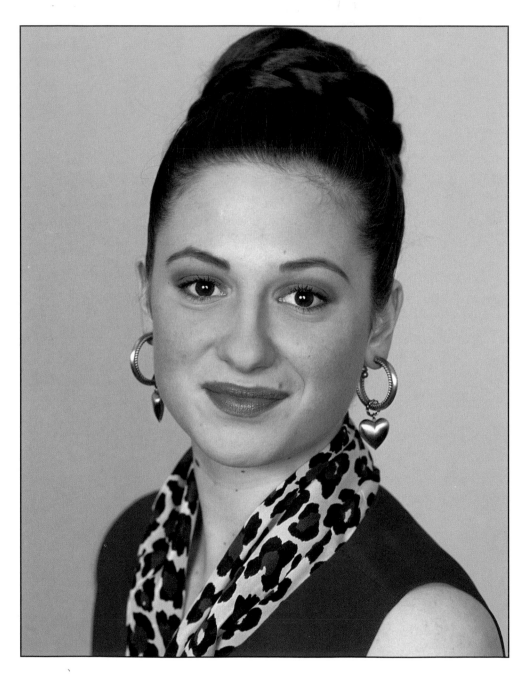

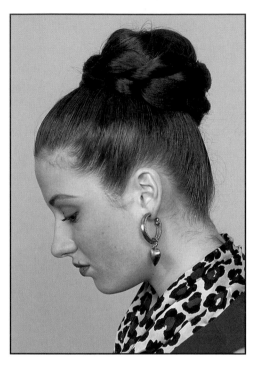

*h*ere's how to make an ordinary bun extraordinary. The basic twisting and coiling motion used to create the Topknot (see page 17) is also used for this High-Volume Topknot. Unlike the basic Topknot, however, which is coiled several times around the ponytail, the High-Volume Topknot is coiled only once. For a loose, high-volume look, you must use your fingers to fan, or spread, out the hair of the ponytail.

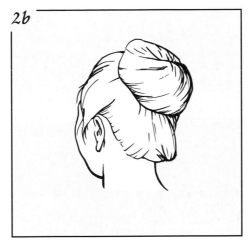

2a

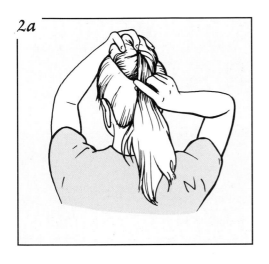

2b

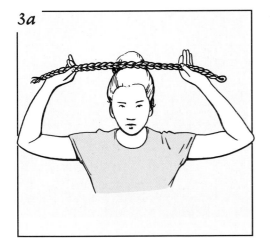

3a

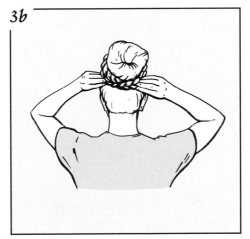

3b

A braided switch, a fake hairpiece, provides extra drama. Although this style is easy enough for beginners, it can be an elegant and dressy look for special occasions.

MATERIALS

covered elastic band
braided switch
hairpins

DIRECTIONS

1. Pull all your hair straight back into a ponytail at the crown of your head. Secure with an elastic band.

2. (**a**) Gently twist the first half-turn of the bun into a loose coil, fanning with your fingers to keep fullness in the hair.

(**b**) Twist the remaining hair an additional half-turn to complete the bun.

3. Place the center of a braided switch at the front of the topknot (**a**). Wrap the braid around the topknot, crisscross the braid in back, and tuck in the ends (**b**).

4. Secure the braid with hairpins along the bottom edge. You may want to add decorative bows or hair ornaments which can also help hide imperfections, if desired.

WRAPAROUND TOPKNOT WITH THREE-STRAND BRAID

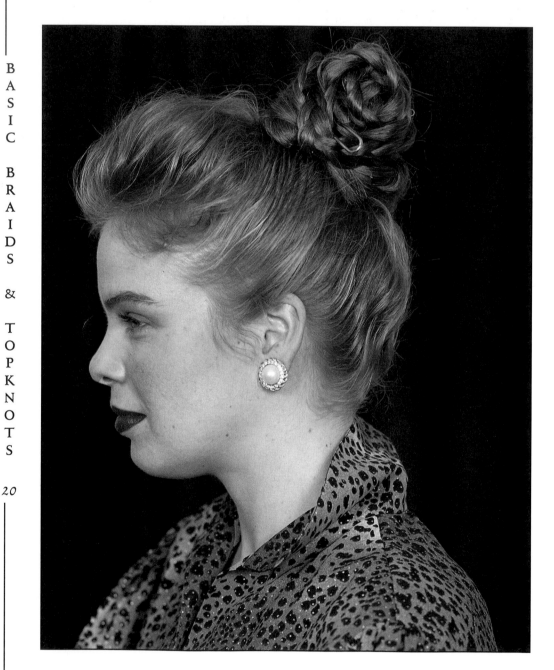

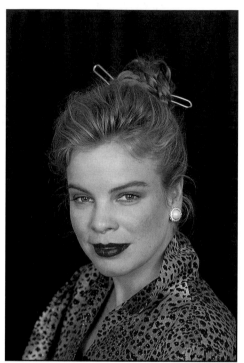

*t*his style starts with a simple bun. Braided strands from a switch are then wrapped around it in order to give the illusion of extra-long hair. The result is a look that can go anywhere—from a country picnic to a city dinner.

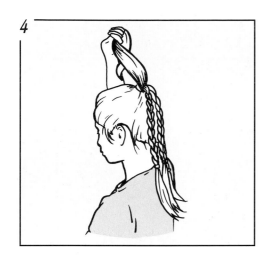

4

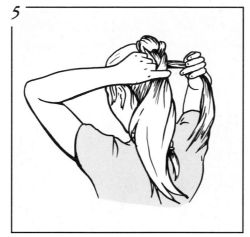

5

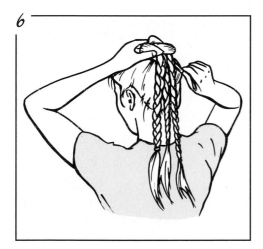

6

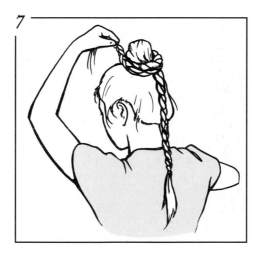

7

4. Lay the switch so that it straddles your ponytail (two braids falling to one side of the ponytail and one on the other). Attach the switch securely with bobby pins under the ponytail.

5. Braid your ponytail. If your ponytail is too short to braid, simply twist it several times and proceed as if it were braided.

6. Twist and coil the braided ponytail into a bun. Pin to secure.

7. One by one, wrap the braids from the switch around the bun and pin securely. Play with your own variations as you wrap, forming loops if desired. If you have trouble with short pieces sticking out, try wrapping the long braids of the switch over them to hide them.

8. Add hair ornaments, if desired.

MATERIALS

switch
hairpins   bobby pins
covered elastic band

DIRECTIONS

1. Divide the switch into three sections. Braid each section for three long narrow braids.

2. Section off some of your own hair above your forehead, tease for height as desired, and pin back at crown. This step not only adds height, but also helps keep shorter strands in place.

3. Gather the rest of your hair up into a high ponytail and secure with a covered elastic band.

FRENCH BRAIDS

❖ ❖ ❖

BASIC LOOSE FRENCH BRAID

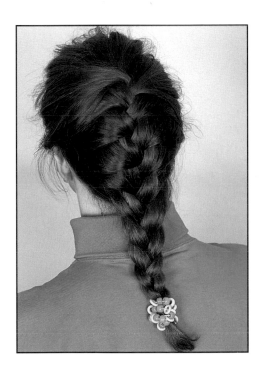 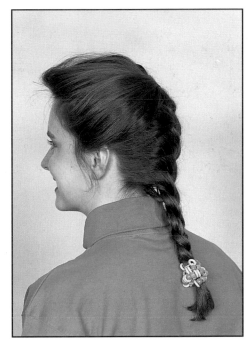 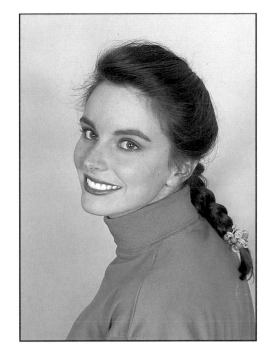

*O*nce you've mastered basic braiding, you are ready for the next step— classic French braiding. The technique is the same as for basic braiding except that you work in new strands of hair from alongside the braid as you plait. This loose version makes learning fun and easy—the strands of hair are large and they are taken only from the back of the head. Later you'll learn to plait tightly and to pull strands from the sides of the head around to the back. You'll use this style for more than just learning—it's sure to become a staple of your hairdressing wardrobe.

MATERIALS

covered elastic band
bow or hair ornament

DIRECTIONS

1. To begin, section off hair from the front, crown, and sides of the head; leave the back to be worked in shortly.

2. Divide this section into 3 strands, and begin to braid them.

3. When you are ready to work the left strand into the braid again, add to it first by picking up loose hair from alongside the braid.

4. Add to the right strand similarly. Repeat steps 3 and 4, alternating sides and adding hair as you braid.

5. When you reach the nape of the neck, continue working a basic braid to the end of the hair and secure with an elastic band. Cover the elastic with a bow or other hair ornament.

PRACTICE TIPS

Professionals like to use their pinkie to pick up the strands from the side. This way, they can continue to hold the braid securely with their other fingers. Each new strand they pick up is about the same size, which keeps the main braid even and neat. For neat sectioning, drag your pinkie fingernail across the scalp in a straight line from the ear to the braid. Your fingernail will function much like the tooth of a comb to make an even part.

For a tighter braid, pull down on individual strands as you braid them. Using smaller strands will also help to create a tighter braid. The loose look shown here uses large sections. With a little practice, you will be able to control the amount of tightness you want. In any case, try to maintain consistent tension throughout so the braid has a uniform appearance from top to bottom.

1
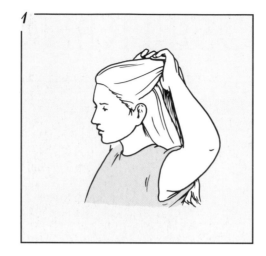

2
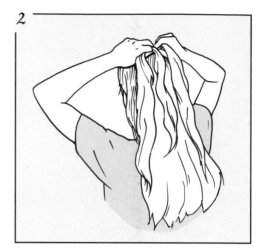

3
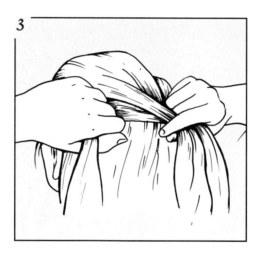

4
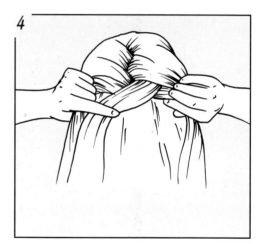

5
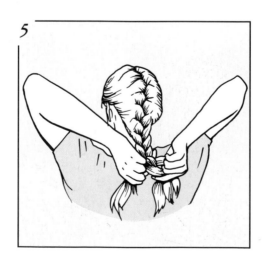

BASIC FRENCH BRAID

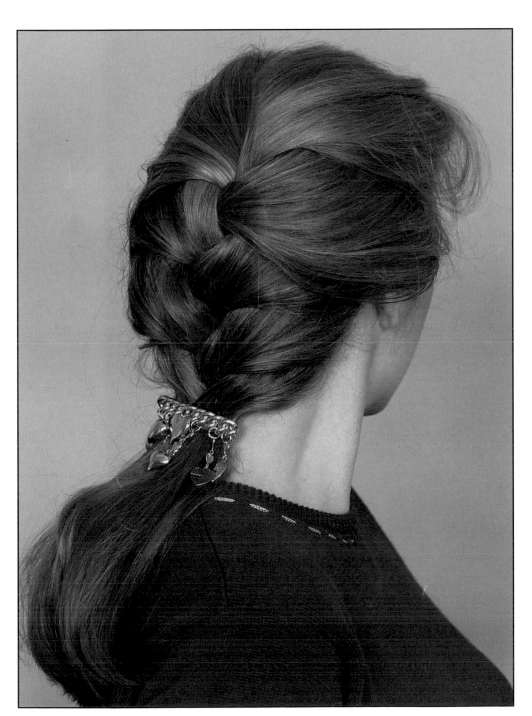

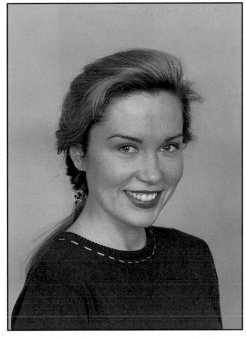

*t*he Basic French Braid is the same as the Basic Loose French Braid except for the first and last steps. The loose version is easier for beginners, so you may want to practice it a few times before trying this one.

MATERIALS
....

covered elastic band
hair ornament

DIRECTIONS

1. To begin, section off hair from the front and crown only; leave the sides and back loose to work in shortly.

2. Divide this section into 3 strands (**a**) and begin to braid them (**b**).

3. When you are ready to work the left strand into the braid again, add to it first by picking up loose hair from alongside the braid.

4. Add to the right strand similarly. Repeat steps 3 and 4, alternating sides and adding hair as you braid.

5. Secure the braid at the nape of the neck with a covered elastic band. Add the hair ornament of your choice.

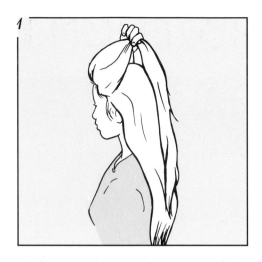

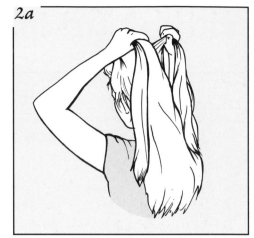

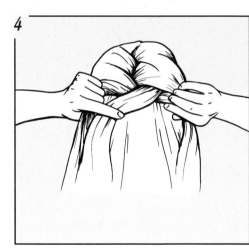

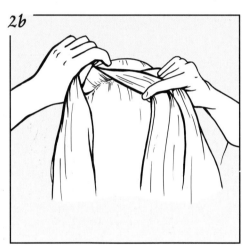

FRENCH BRAID ROLLED UNDER

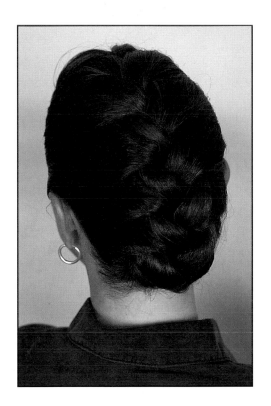

MATERIALS

covered elastic band
hairpins

DIRECTIONS

1–4. Work the Basic French Braid steps 1–4.

5. End the French braid and begin a regular braid slightly above the nape of the neck. Allow greater space above the nape if you have very long or very thick hair. Tie a covered elastic band around bottom end.

6. Fold the end up under the braid and pin in place.

*R*olling a French braid under gives your hair a much more polished look than the Basic French Braid, yet it is really no more difficult to do. While this style is striking in its simplicity, it also lends itself to spicing up with decoration. Add flowers for a romantic look or whimsical ornaments for fun. In the office or for an evening out, this is a lovely way to keep your hair off your neck in the heat of the summer.

5
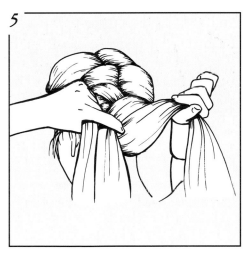

6
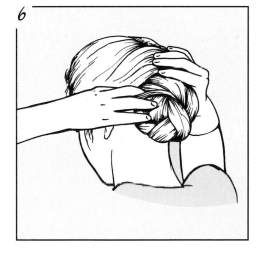

FRENCH BRAIDS ON THE SIDES

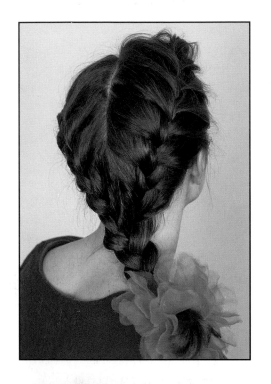

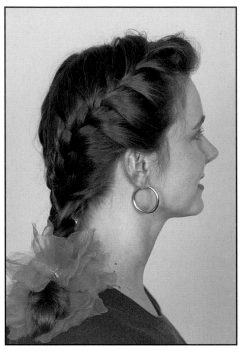

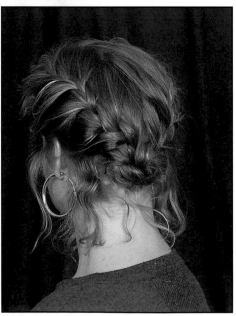

*O*nce you've mastered basic French braiding, you can easily create side braids like these. This style works especially well with fine hair. There are even two versions, one for long hair, the other for medium-length hair. Notice how the looser tension on the shorter version relaxes the style. Practically any braid can appear more casual by loosening it. Simply pull gently on small sections of hair with the end of a rat tail comb. This technique can also improve the braid if it is uneven due to irregular tension during braiding.

MATERIALS

covered elastic band   hairpins
hair ornament

FOR LONG HAIR

DIRECTIONS

1. Part hair in front as desired, ending at the center of the crown. Then continue the part straight down the center of the back of the head.

2. Work one side at a time. To begin, clip one section off to the side, out of the way. Divide the hair on the working side into 3 sections and plait as you would for a Basic French Braid **(a)**. Pull extra strands from either side of the braid, drawing hair away from the face and away from the part. When you reach the neck **(b)**, secure with a clip.

3. Plait the opposite side in the same way. When French braids meet at the nape of the neck, combine the hair. Divide the combined hair into three strands and continue with a Basic Braid. Secure the end with a covered elastic and cover with ribbon tied in a bow.

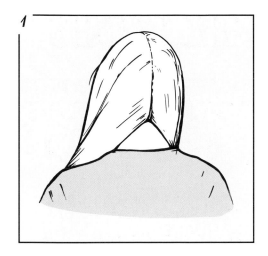

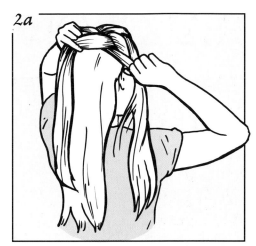

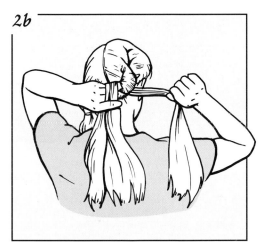

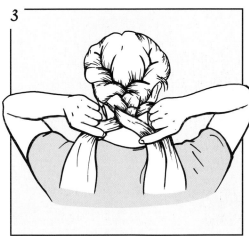

FOR MEDIUM-LENGTH HAIR

DIRECTIONS

1. Part hair in front as desired, ending at the center of the crown. Then continue the part straight down the center of the back of the head. Cover with a hair ornament.

2. Work one side at a time. To begin, clip one section off to the side, out of the way. Divide the hair on the working side into 3 sections and plait as you would for a Basic French Braid. Pull extra strands from either side of the braid, drawing hair away from the face and away from the part (**a**). Secure with a clip (**b**) and plait opposite side.

3. Continue each French braid by working a Basic Braid until you reach end of hair. Crisscross these two braids at nape of neck and pin to secure. Short ends can be tucked into braid. Use gel if necessary to tame flyaway ends.

INVERTED CROWN DOWN

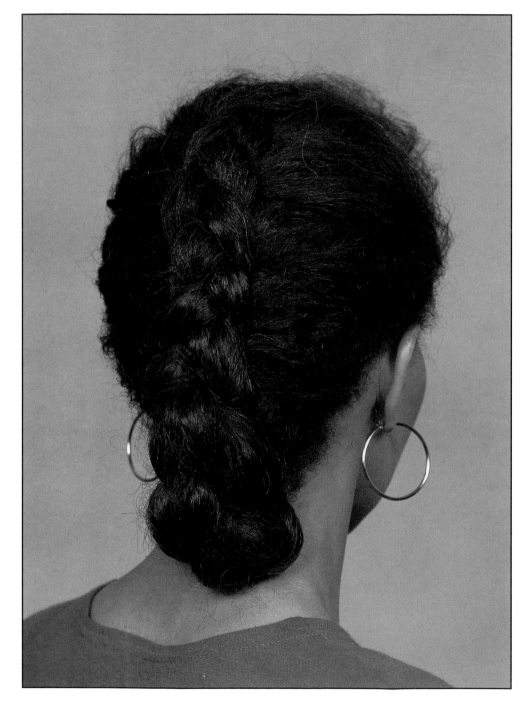

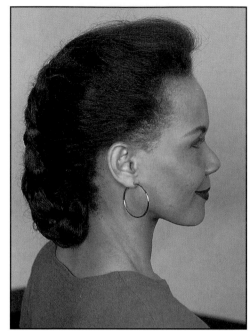

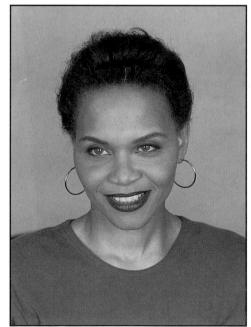

*t*he Inverted Crown Down French braid is similar to the Basic Loose French Braid, except the strands are crossed under instead of over as they are plaited. The resulting braid has an unusual and intricate appearance that's sure to attract attention. It is a little tricky, but once you've mastered the Basic Loose French Braid, you should be able to get this one down with a little practice. It makes a wonderfully different style for special occasions.

MATERIALS

covered elastic band
hairpins

DIRECTIONS

1. To begin, section off hair at the front, crown, and sides of the head. (The back will be worked in shortly.)

2. Divide this section into three strands. Begin to braid, crossing right strand *under* the center strand, then crossing left strand *under* the center.

3. When you are ready to work a right strand into the braid again, add to it first by picking up loose hair from alongside the braid. Remember to cross the right strand under the center strand to maintain the distinctive inverted appearance.

4. Add to the left strand similarly. Repeat steps 3 and 4, alternating sides and adding hair as you braid.

5. From just above the nape of the neck to the end of the hair, continue working in the Basic Braid, but pass the outside strands under rather than over the center strand. Secure the end with a covered elastic band. Fold the braid under and pin it in position at the nape of the neck.

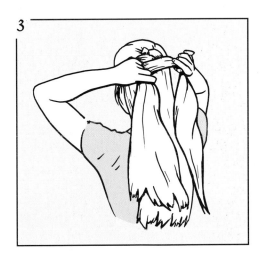

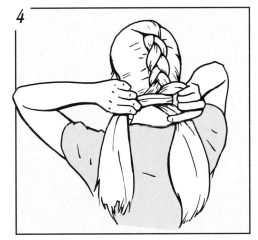

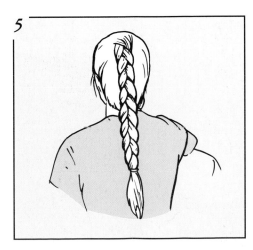

FRENCH-BRAIDED HAIRBAND

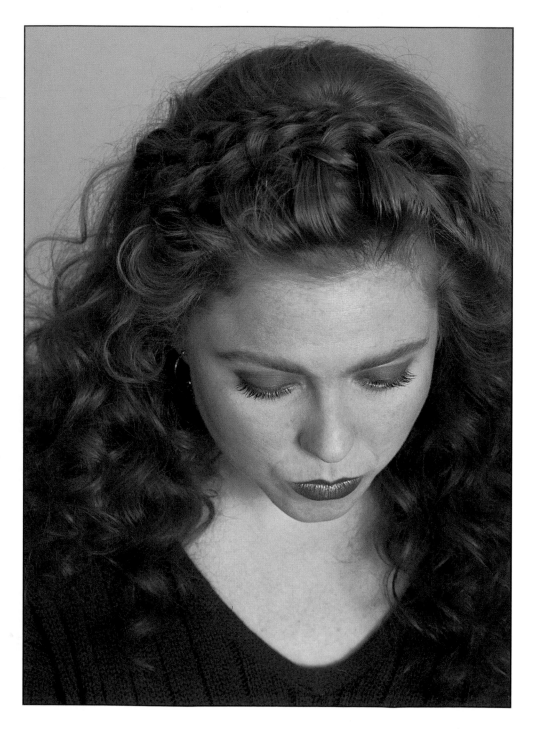

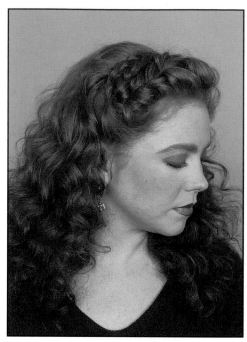

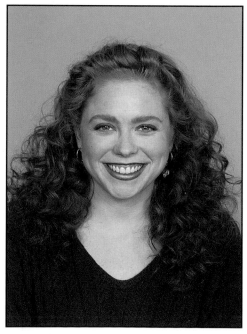

*i*f you've already learned to French braid, you'll enjoy this easy variation. It's a French braid across the top, folded back on itself. Perfect for curly hair, it acts as a sort of "natural" hairband for the rest of the hair, which is left loose and flowing.

MATERIALS

covered elastic band
hairpins

DIRECTIONS

1. Part hair from ear to ear, across the top of the head. Clip the loose hair back to hold it away from the working area.

2. Sweep the entire front section of hair across the top of the head. Starting from the left ear, brush up, sweep across the top, and let the entire section of hair fall down to the right ear.

3. Begin French braiding at the left ear and continue across the top of the head to the right ear.

4. Work a Basic Braid to the end of the hair and fasten with a covered elastic band.

5. Wrap the Basic Braid back over the top of your head, alongside the French braid. Tuck the ends into the French braid. Secure with hairpins. Loosen the front, if needed, with the end of a rat tail comb. Fluff up the hair in back for volume.

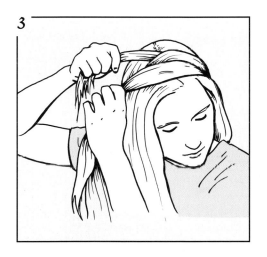

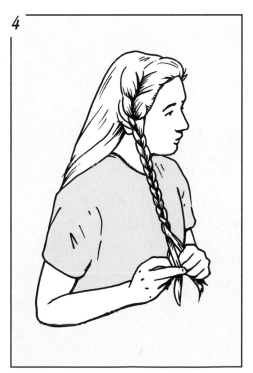

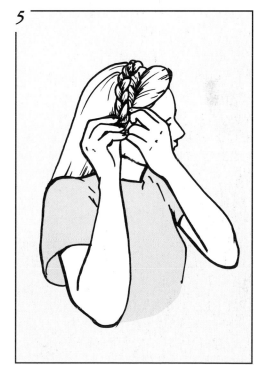

FISHTAIL

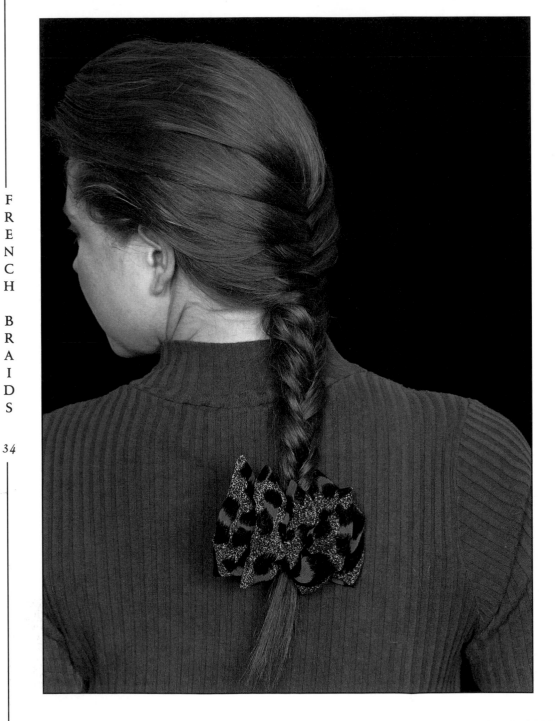

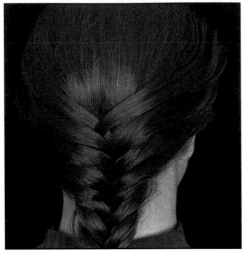

*t*he pretty shimmering fishtail looks best on straight, healthy hair. The "weave" allows the hair to catch the light from many directions, giving it a radiant quality. For an evening out, you can highlight the design with rhinestones (packets of rhinestones are available in notions departments). Glue them to hairpins and insert the hairpins here and there throughout the braid.

MATERIALS

covered elastic band
hair ornament

DIRECTIONS

1. Brush all hair straight back. To begin, section off two small strands of hair, one from the left temple and one from the right. Each section should be about 1 inch (2.5cm) thick.

2. Cross the strands of hair from these two sections, right over left, at the back of the head.

3. Hold the crossed strands in place by pressing them flat with your right hand. With your left hand, take up a new section of hair from directly underneath the previous left section. Make sure it is similar in size.

4. Cross the new left section over the right strand most recently added and hold in place, pressed flat, with your left hand.

5. With your right hand, take up a new section of hair from the right side of the head. Cross the new right section over the left strand most recently added and hold it in place, pressed flat, with your right hand.

6. Repeat steps 3 through 5 until the Fishtail reaches the nape of the neck.

7. Continue working the fishtail pattern, pulling strands of hair from the underside of the "ponytail" and crossing them at the center. (Although the hair hasn't been gathered into an elastic band, it will fall like a ponytail down the back.)

8. Secure the end with a covered elastic band. Add a hair ornament, if desired.

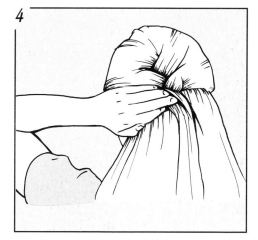

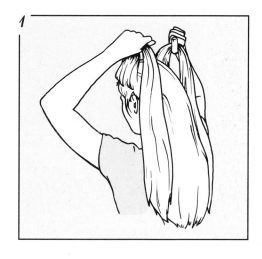

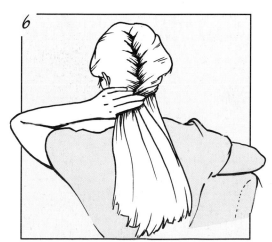

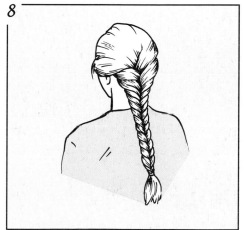

Chapter Three

ROPE BRAIDS

❖ ❖ ❖

5. Transfer both strands to your right hand, using your fingers to keep the strands crossed, separated, and twisted. (Try holding one strand between your ring finger and middle finger and the other between your middle finger and index finger.) Clench your hand tightly, pinching strands to prevent untwisting. Using your left hand, section off some new hair as before. Twist this new strand (**C**), then carry it under the bottom strand (**A**) and over the top strand (**B**). Switch hands, combine strands A and B into one strand, then transfer the 2 remaining strands to your right hand.

6. Repeat steps 4 and 5 until you reach the nape of the neck. Secure with a clip.

7. Rope-braid hair on the other side of the part in a similar manner, following steps 2 through 6 and reversing directions for left and right.

8. Combine the ends of both braids at the nape of the neck and secure with a hair clip, letting loose hair below clip fall in a ponytail.

9. Add bow or hair ornament, if desired.

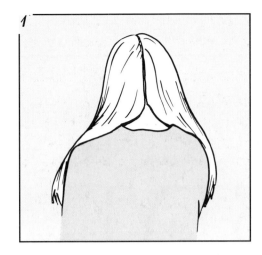

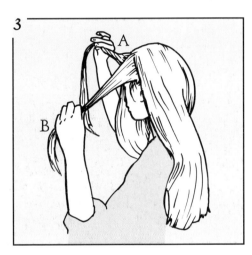

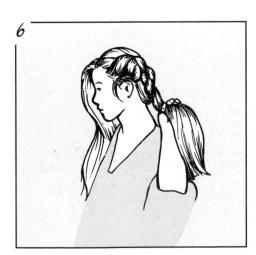

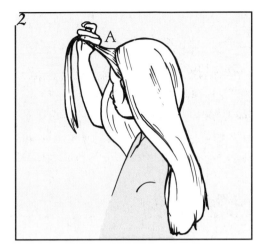

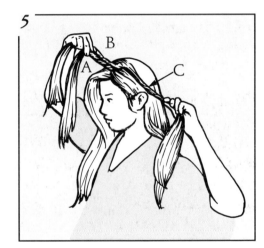

Chapter Four

EVENING STYLES

◆ ◆ ◆

French Twist

Coronet

Chignon

French Braids with Ribbon

Free Spirit

Crimping

Upside-Down French Braid

FRENCH TWIST

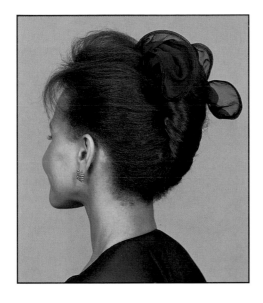

W ith a little practice you can easily master the simple technique for creating this timeless style. While it's not actually a braid, we felt that no hair book would be complete without the classic French twist. Its upward sweep and sleek lines make one appear thinner by adding height and accentuating the length of the neck. The graceful curve complements the most sophisticated eveningwear, yet it is versatile enough to look appropriate in the boardroom as well as in the ballroom.

MATERIALS

hairpins

DIRECTIONS

1. Gather all of your hair back as you would for a ponytail. (Do not bind with an elastic band.)

2. Twist counterclockwise about three times until hair feels tight.

3. Hold the twist in your right hand. Place your left thumb along the back of your head and wrap the twist around it. Tuck the loose ends into the "seam" and shape as desired.

4. Continue holding in place as you pin loosely but securely with hairpins.

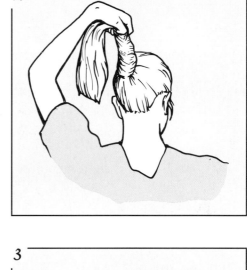

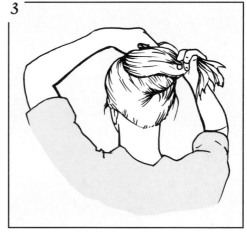

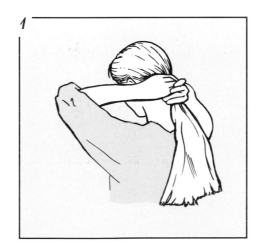

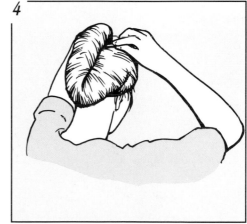

CORONET

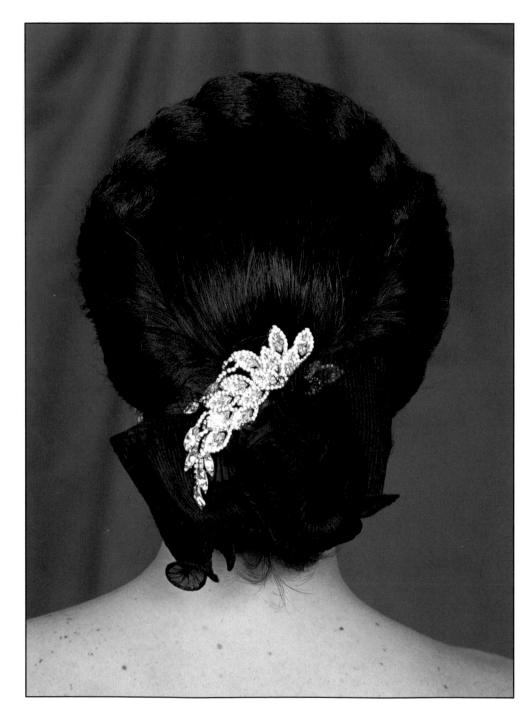

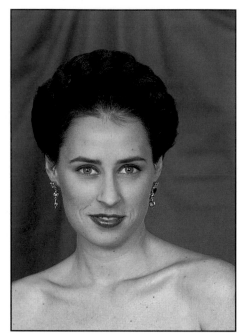

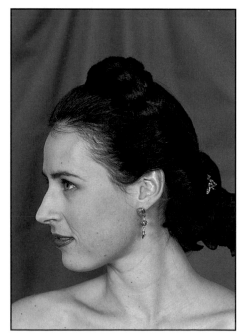

*t*he coronet, a small crown, lends its name to this formal hairstyle. The regal aura is achieved with a braided switch and a few easy-to-follow secrets. While perfect for the most formal evening event, this style would also look stunning with clothing reminiscent of the thirties and forties. Whatever the occasion, it will make you feel like a queen.

MATERIALS

braided switch
hair clips
covered elastic band
bobby pins
hairpins
hair spray
ruched fabric

DIRECTIONS

1. Brush hair straight back. Seperate side sections and clip away from working area.

2. Tease (back-comb) top section and comb back to join hair at back of head. Gather into a ponytail above the nape of the neck and fasten with a covered elastic band.

3. Lightly spray with hair spray. The finished look should be very neat and orderly.

4. Lay a braided switch across the top of your head, headband style. Wrap the ends around your head so they meet in back, under the ponytail.

5. Pin securely at the back with bobby pins. Add about six more pins around the base of switch coronet to hold it securely.

6. Tease one side piece. Spray lightly with hair spray. Comb back and fold this section of hair over the braid. Twist and tuck the ends of this side section of hair into the inner circle formed by the braid, completely covering that entire section of braid. Secure with hairpins along inside edge of braid.

7. Repeat on other side.

8. Cover elastic with ruched fabric. Fold ponytail over the bottom section of the braid. Tuck under and pin to secure. Add hair ornaments as desired to complete the "crown."

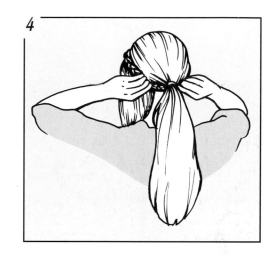

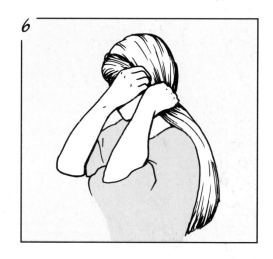

CHIGNON

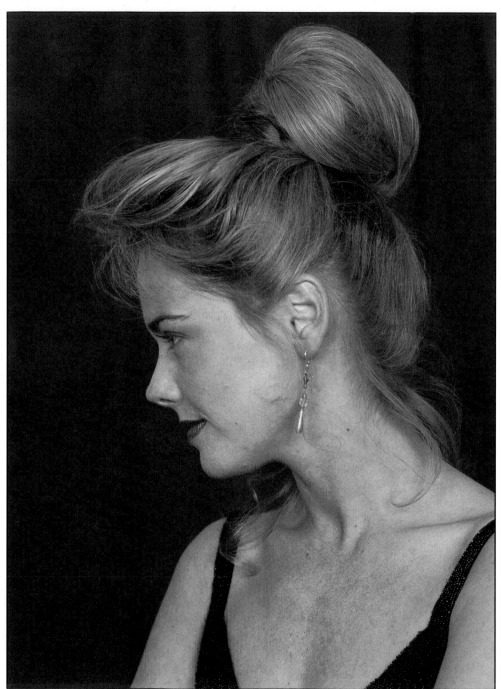

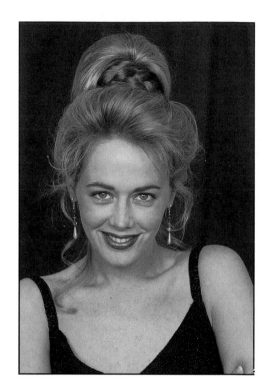

*t*he chignon, French for "bun," is an *irresistible combination of softness and elegance. You can add to the romantic look by leaving some tendrils to curl around the face and the nape of the neck. This chignon gains volume by using a switch, but some extra teasing can produce similar results. Another trick is to stick two or three bobby pins into the center of the ponytail to create a framework for more height.*

MATERIALS

braided switch (if desired)
covered elastic band
hairpins

DIRECTIONS

1. Part the hair from ear to ear across the top of the head and let it fall forward. Gather the remaining hair into a ponytail on top of the head and secure with a thick covered elastic band.

2. Tease (back-comb) the entire front section, including sides, to add body. Sweep the teased hair back to the ponytail, twist once, and wrap end around the ponytail elastic. Fasten with hairpins. You can leave some tendrils to hang and/or curl, if desired.

3. If using a switch:
Fasten it to the ponytail elastic, then wrap it around the ponytail. Tuck in ends and pin. Tease the ponytail hair. Fan out the hair and fold it over the switch at the sides and back. Gently tuck ends into the bottom outside edge of the braid and fasten with hairpins.

4. If not using a switch:
(a) Section off a medium-sized strand of hair from the underside of the ponytail. Braid hair to the end, then wrap around elastic band. Secure the end of the braid with a bobby pin underneath the ponytail.

(b) Tease ponytail hair to create more volume. Fan hair out from center and fold it under itself, securing with hairpins all around the base of bun.

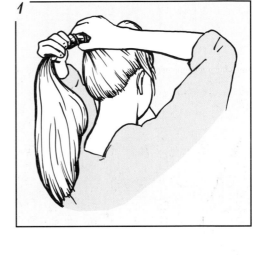

1

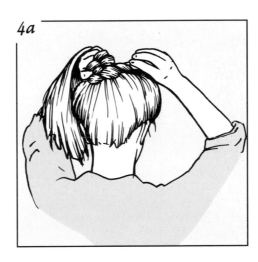

4a

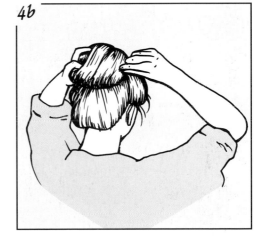

4b

FRENCH BRAIDS WITH RIBBON

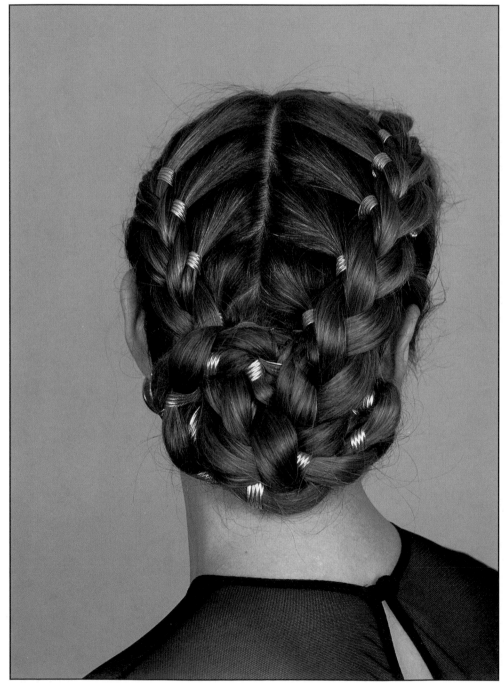

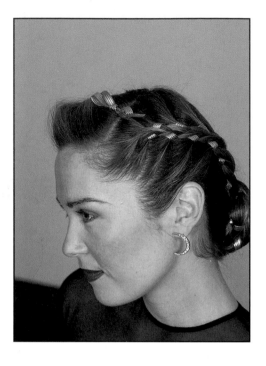

*W*hat's the secret to success for this intricate, special-occasion style? Ask a friend to do the braiding and keep sections small, tight, and even. You'll need ribbon for this style; metallic ribbons add a shimmery quality and tend to stay in place better than satin ribbons. Once the braider gets the rhythm of the technique, it goes fairly quickly. The finished results are well worth the effort.

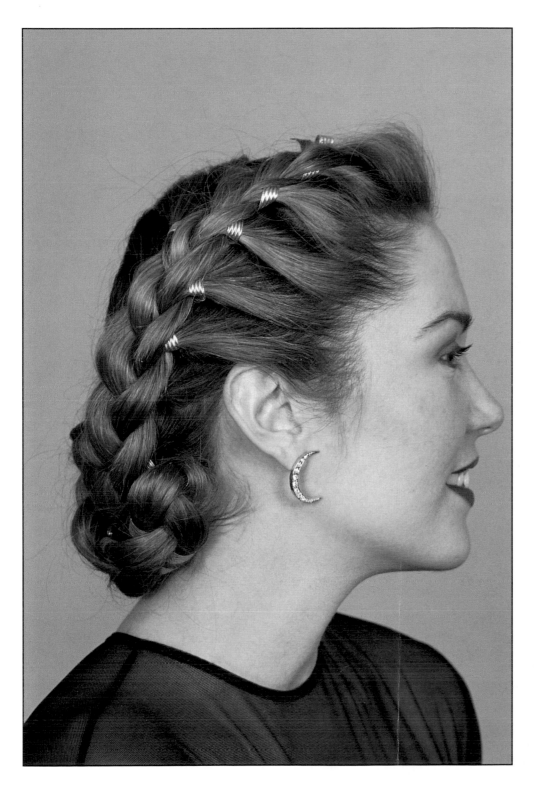

MATERIALS

2 1-yard (1m) lengths narrow ribbon
covered elastic band
bobby pins

DIRECTIONS

1. Part the hair diagonally in front,
beginning at the side and angling
back 45 degrees toward the center of
the crown. From there, continue the
part straight down the center of the
back of the head.

2. Working one side of the head
at a time, you will proceed with a
French braid. Keep the sections tiny,
tight, and close to the head. To
begin, lay one of the lengths of
ribbon under the first section,
leaving a 6-inch (15cm) extension at
the top. As the braid is formed, wrap
the ribbon *under* each newly added
section. This will allow the ribbon
to be caught up in the braiding,
moving from side to side, back and
forth across the braid.

3. When you reach the nape of the
neck, continue a regular braid and
work the ribbon back and forth by
wrapping it *under* the strand that is
being crossed each time. Secure the
end with a covered elastic band.

4. Repeat steps 2 and 3 to braid the hair on the other side of the head.

5. Cross braids at nape of neck (a) and fold each one into center, pinning neatly with bobby pins (b). Tie the top lengths of ribbon into a bow.

1
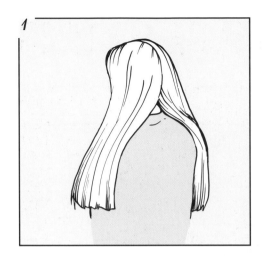

2
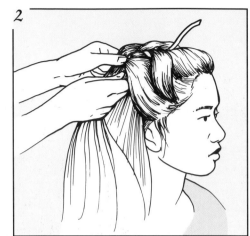

3
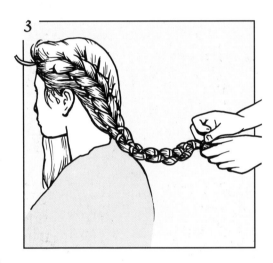

5a
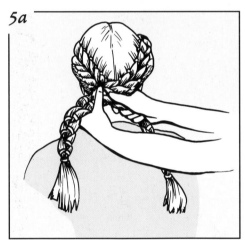

5b
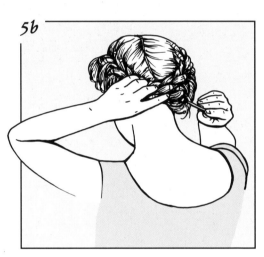

FREE SPIRIT

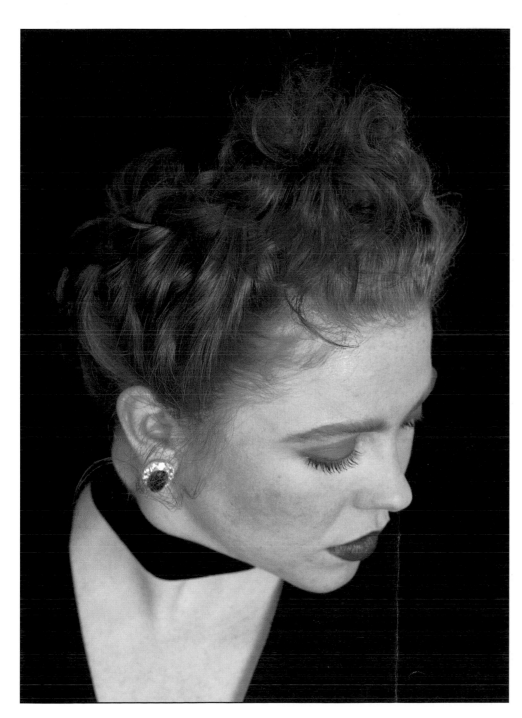

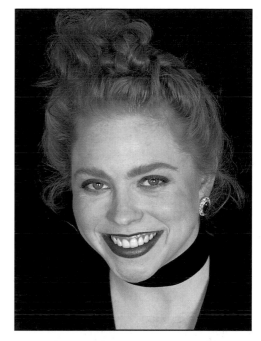

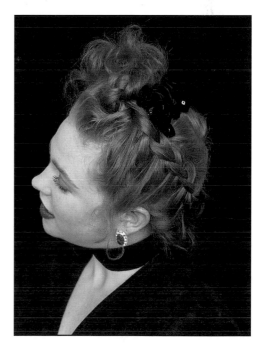

ooking for something really unusual? Try a zigzag part, add French braiding that goes from back to front, and finish by leaving the ends to dangle loose on top. This style defies tradition at every step— it is only for the brave at heart!

MATERIALS

rat tail comb
hair clip
covered elastic bands
hairpins

DIRECTIONS

1. Use a rat tail comb to make a zig zag part down the middle of the head, both on top and down the back. Clip one section off to the side as you work the other side.

2. Begin French braiding behind your ear, working up toward the top of the head. Keep the braid centered in the section. When you reach your forehead, continue with a regular braid to the end of the hair, leaving a "tail" hanging in your face. Secure the end with a covered elastic band.

3. Repeat step 2 to braid the hair on the other side of the head.

4. Tie the two braids in a knot and pin in place. Fluff out the loose ends to create a whimsical curly top. (If you don't have naturally curly hair, you can use a curling iron on these ends.)

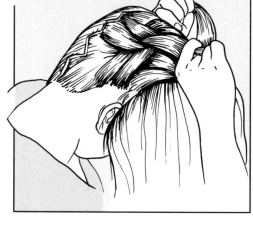

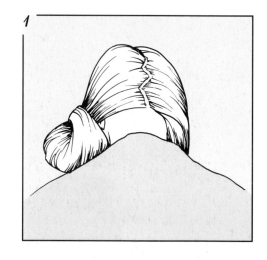

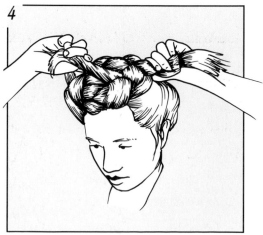

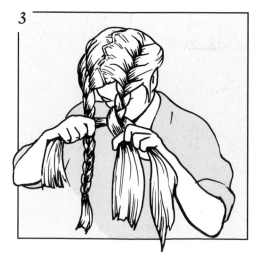

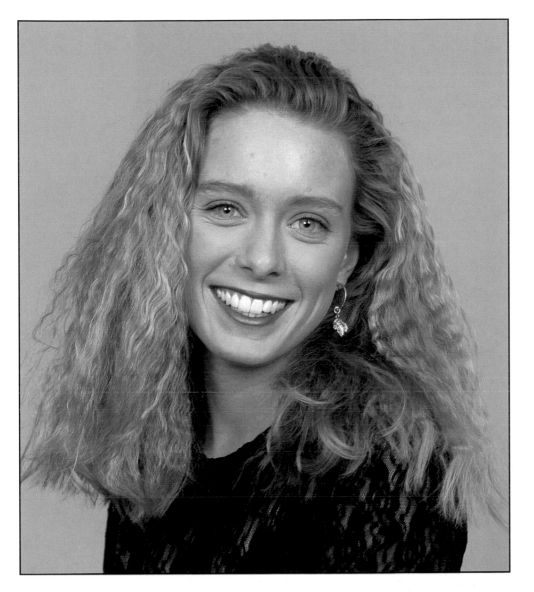

CRIMPING

MATERIALS

hair clip
covered elastic bands

DIRECTIONS

1. Gather and clip your hair on top of your head.

2. Beginning at the nape of the neck, take a small section of hair and braid it, spritzing with water from a spray bottle as you work. Secure end with a covered elastic band. Take up new sections for braiding in uneven rows, letting hair down from clip as needed. Braid the top of the head last. Braid away from face.

3. When entire head is braided (about 24 braids for average hair thickness), allow hair to dry naturally or use a hair dryer.

4. When hair is dry, unravel all the braids. If a hair dryer is used, allow hair to cool before taking out the braids.

*C*rimped hair results from braiding damp hair. When the braids are dry and unraveled, the hair has a spirit all its own—wild and sexy. Use this trick on hot summer days: it's late afternoon and you've just come home from swimming. You quickly braid your damp hair (well, as quickly as you can make twenty-four braids). You feel so much cooler, and by the time the sun goes down, you're ready to unravel your hair and go out dancing. Remember not to make the rows of braids too even or they will separate after the hair is combed out.

UPSIDE-DOWN FRENCH BRAID

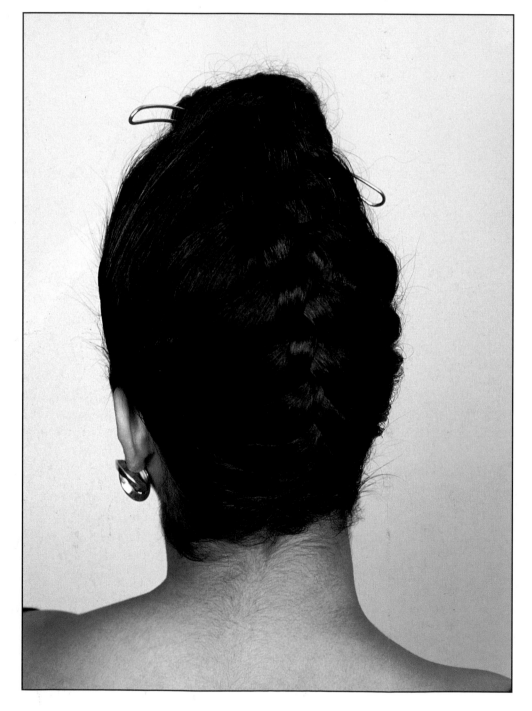

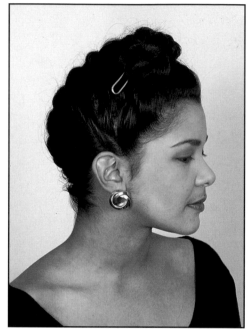

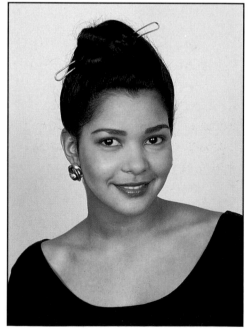

*t*his French braid starts at the neck, travels neatly up the back of the head, and ends in a topknot in front. You have to bend over, brush your hair down, and work upside-down to achieve this unique braid. A very sophisticated and polished look, it's only for those with advanced skill… or a helpful friend.

MATERIALS

covered elastic band
hairpins

DIRECTIONS

1. Bend over and brush hair forward.

2. With head tilted forward, begin French-braiding small sections at the nape of the neck (**2a**). At the top of the ear, begin taking triangular sections. Take bigger sections as you approach the center of the top of the head (**2b**).

3. When all the hair is gathered into the French braid, continue to work to ends of hair in a basic braid.

Secure with a covered elastic band. The basic braid should start in the center of the top of the head.

4. Stand up straight, holding the braid straight up (**4a**). Roll the braid forward onto itself and down to the top of the head, forming a topknot (**4b**). Pin to secure.

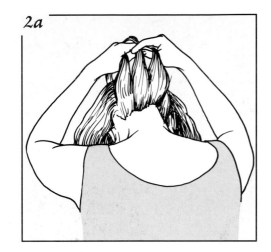

2a

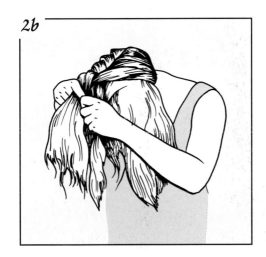

2b

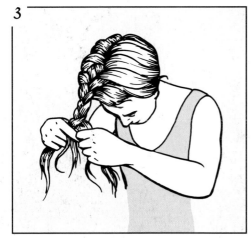

3

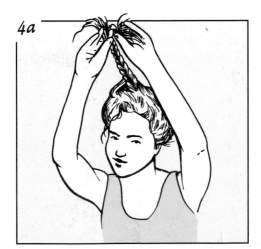

4a

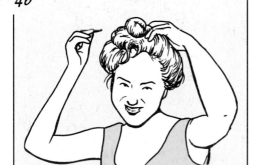

4b

Chapter Five

BRAIDS
FOR
KIDS

❖ ❖ ❖

Heidi Braids

Rainbow Braids

Triple Clip Braid

HEIDI BRAIDS

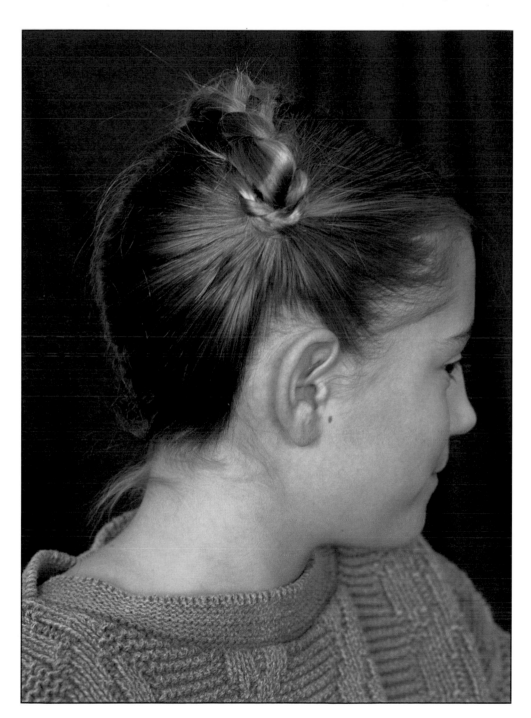

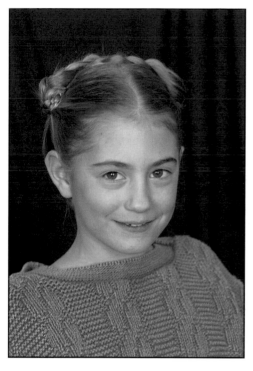

*M*ost little girls love to play with their hair. As they experiment, they discover how hairstyles can change their appearance while learning some of the basics of good grooming.

Here's a style that will make your little one feel special and also look very cute. Named for the famous children's book, this hairdo recalls Heidi's wholesome yet distinct style.

MATERIALS

covered elastic band
hairpins

DIRECTIONS

1. Part hair in the middle across top
and down back of head. Make two
pigtails, one over each ear, and
secure with covered elastic bands.

2. Braid the pigtails and secure the
ends with elastic bands.

3. Crisscross the braids on top of
the head and fasten with hairpins.

4. Wrap loose hair at the end of
each braid around the exposed
pigtail elastics.

5. The elastics at the end of the
pigtails can be hidden by tucking
them under the the braids and
pinning.

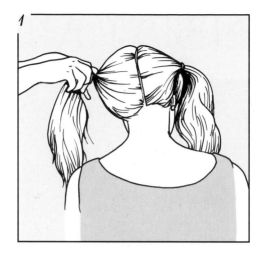

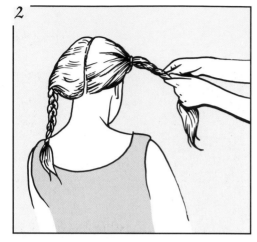

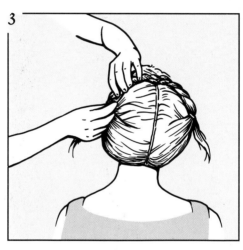

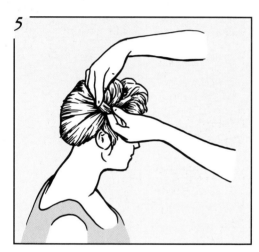

RAINBOW BRAIDS

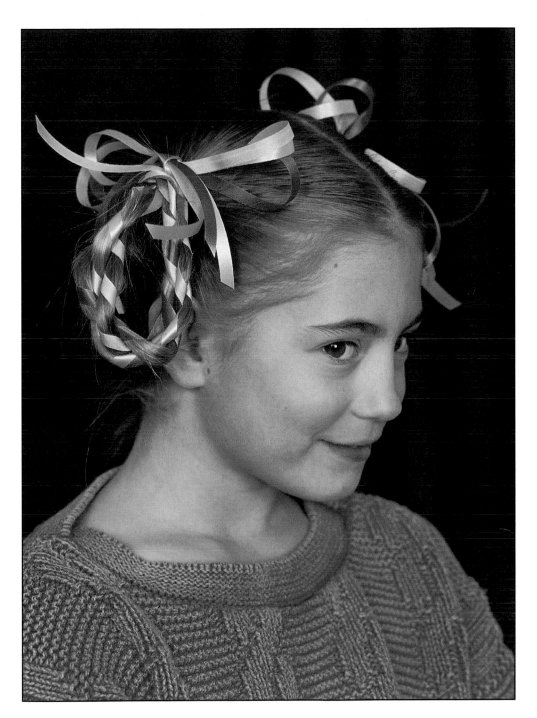

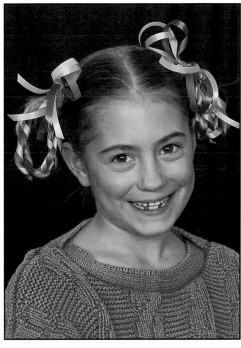

*t*his colorful style will make its wearer really stand out, so it's not for shrinking violets! It's a fun look with a lot of personality. You'll need six ribbons in your little girl's favorite colors. Match her outfit or use the whole rainbow! You're sure to have fun shopping together for different ribbons, choosing extra shades for special outfits and occasions.

MATERIALS

6 ribbons, each 1 yard (1m) long
covered elastic bands
hair clips

DIRECTIONS

1. Part hair in the middle across top and down back of head. Make 2 pigtails, one over each ear, and secure with covered elastic bands.

2. Pull 3 ribbons through each elastic band. Leave about 12 inches (30cm) of each ribbon free at the top.

3. Divide one pigtail into 3 strands. Wrap each strand of hair with a ribbon streamer and clip each end.

4. Braid to the end of the hair, remove the clips, and secure with an elastic band.

5. Repeat steps 3 and 4 to braid other pigtail.

6. Turn each braid under, joining the ribbons from the bottom of the braid with the ribbons at the top of the braid to form a loop. Tie ribbons into bows.

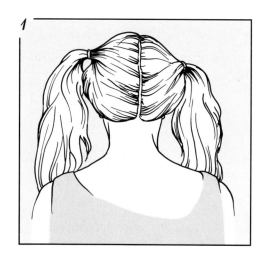

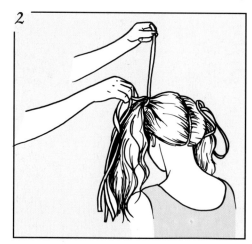

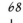

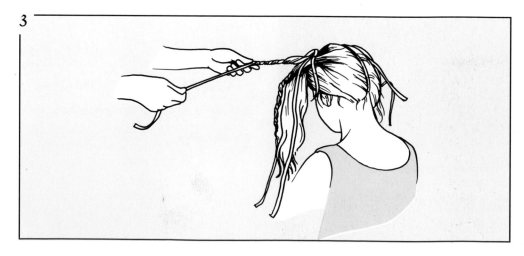

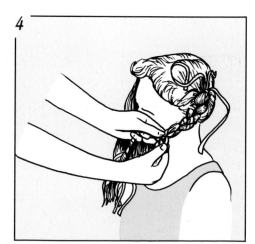

TRIPLE CLIP BRAID

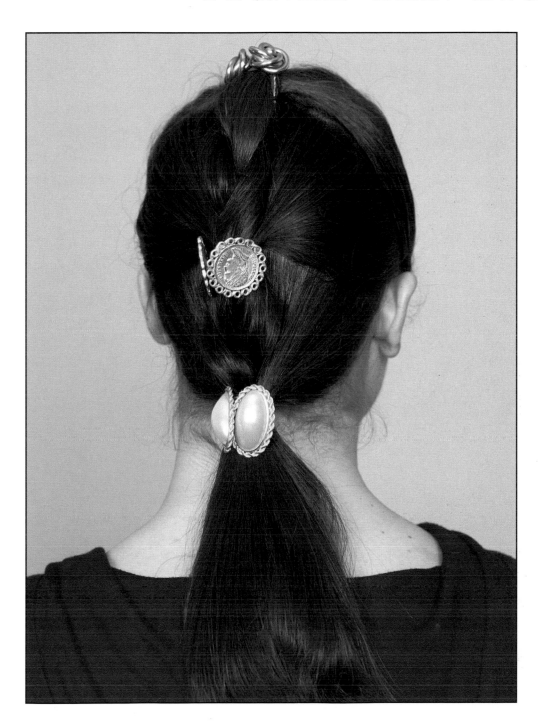

*S*o many different hair ornaments are available today—the hardest part about the Triple Clip Braid is choosing which ones you like the best! Ornaments that are already attached to elastics are the easiest to use in this style. If you feel creative, you can also try making your own. Attach small unbreakable tree ornaments to covered elastics for the holidays or add flowers from your garden for spring and summer styles.

It's fun to build a collection of hair treasures—they make great birthday party favors or rewards for good grades.

MATERIALS

covered elastic bands
3 hair ornaments

DIRECTIONS

1. Sweep hair from sides and front into a ponytail at the crown of the head. Fasten with a covered elastic band and decorate with a hair ornament.

2. Braid the ponytail to the center of the back of the head.

3. Gather the hair from both sides of the braid and join with braid in an elastic band. Once again, decorate with a hair ornament.

4. Gather remaining hair in a ponytail at nape of neck. Secure with an elastic band and add a third ornament.

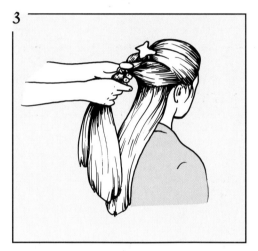
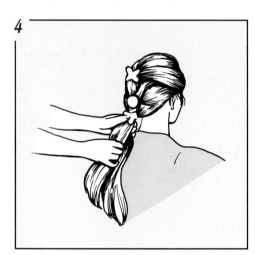
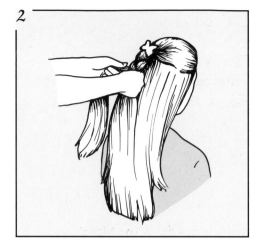
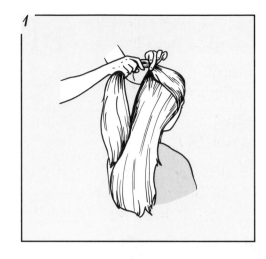

CREDITS

(Wraparound Topknot with
Three-Strand Braid)
Hair ornaments by Bradley Johns

(Basic Loose French Braid)
Hair clip by Kirk's Folly

(Basic French Braid)
Hair ornament by Debra Moises

(French Braids on the Sides)
Hair accessory by Debra Moises

(French-Braided Hairband)
Earrings by Kirk's Folly

(Fishtail)
Hair ornament by Kirk's Folly

(Basic Rope Braid/variation I)
Earrings by Kirk's Folly

(Rope to Bun/version II)
Hair accessory by Debra Moises
Earrings by Kirk's Folly

(Rope to French Braid)
Hair ornament by Kirk's Folly

(Loose Rope Braids)
Bow by Debra Moises

(French Twist)
Hair accessory by Debra Moises

(Coronet)
Earrings and hair ornament by
Kirk's Folly

(Upside-Down French Braid)
Hair ornaments by Bradley Johns

(Triple Clip Braid)
Hair ornaments by Kirk's Folly

SOURCES

Bradley Johns
Available through Orbie at
Elizabeth Arden Salon
691 5th Avenue
New York, NY 10022
(212) 319-3910

Kirk's Folly
389 Fifth Avenue
New York, NY 10016
(212) 683-9797

Debra Moises
1 West 37th Street
New York, NY 10018
(212) 575-4825

INDEX